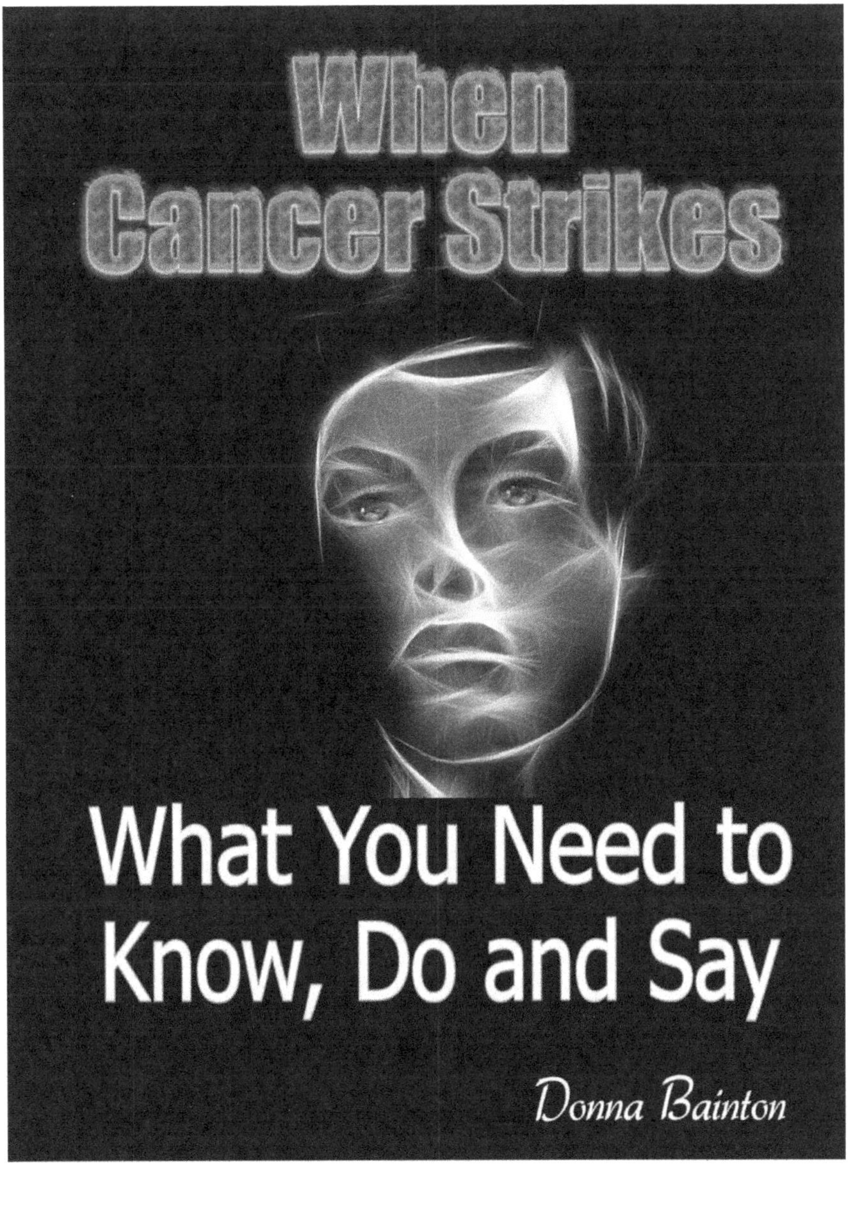

When Cancer Strikes

What You Need to Know, Do and Say

Donna Bainton

Contents

Introduction

It's inevitable. Cancer will touch your life in some way, whether it's as a direct diagnosis or by learning that someone you know has been given the news that they are now dealing with cancer.

As a society we tend to walk through life with an "It's not going to happen to me" attitude in many areas. Cancer is one of them.

So what do you do when you learn that you can no longer live in the land of denial?

How do you handle learning that someone you love is now going to face the cancer battle and all it entails?

The reality is that cancer can strike anyone, not just those who seem to have "high risk factors".

It can be you; it can be your spouse, your mother, your sister or your best friend. It doesn't discriminate, and it's ugly.

In this concise guide we will take you through the process of coping with cancer on a daily basis, and give you some easy-to-use steps that you can follow when someone you love is diagnosed.

- We'll talk about what to expect

- We'll cover your initial reaction, what to say and what not to say

When Cancer Strikes

- We'll give you examples of supportive, yet sensitive things to say to your loved one

- We'll suggest relevant questions, both for you and for your loved one

- We'll give you tips on communication and accountability, coping mechanisms, healing, advocacy, legal matters, and much more

The purpose of this guide is to give you a step-by-step strategy to get you through when the unthinkable happens.

Whether the person fighting cancer is your closest loved one or a casual friend, this guide will help you to know what to say, what to ask and what to do as you face of this frightening diagnosis together.

1: What to Say and What Not to Say

You've just heard the news that someone you care about has cancer. All of the initial reactions and emotions will flood over you. You'll be anxious and scared, angry and feeling helpless.

You won't know what to say to your loved one and, let's face it, there's probably not much you can initially say that will be of any real consequence. She's just been handed devastating news. The emotions she's feeling are the same ones you're experiencing – with the added element that it's happening to her.

At the beginning of this journey the very best thing you can do is to let her know you're there, that you'll help out wherever you can. That might mean driving her to doctor appointments, holding her hand while she undergoes treatment, or just lending an ear when she needs to talk.

Remember that it's OK to talk about feelings as well – both yours and hers.

A common theme with many cancer patients is that they often feel like they're living with the proverbial "elephant in the room."

People are afraid to talk about "The Cancer" and tend to act as though any mention of it if going to cause them to melt into a weeping puddle.

Talk with her about what she wants from you, her expectations and needs, and then follow her wishes.

This may change over time, potentially from week to week, so make sure you leave the lines of communication open.

Don't be afraid to be candid and ask questions, but be sensitive to her emotions.

Pay attention to both verbal and non-verbal cues. It's ok to steer the conversation in a different direction if things start to get too intense for you.

You're going to have to consider your loved one's personality along with the type of relationship you currently have.

Is this a person with whom you are able to talk about most anything or is this someone with whom talk about feelings and personal issues might be awkward and typically less common?

A lot of the literature will tell you to keep your lives as normal as possible and this is one of those areas.

Keep the relationship status quo to some degree… however this might be a good time to bump up the communication style just a wee bit.

Be aware that the first reaction from a new cancer patient is often to cut herself off emotionally. Many people withdraw as a coping mechanism.

Alternatively, she may become very emotional, and may find herself needing your support and presence more than is typical. Both reactions are perfectly normal.

When Cancer Strikes

Sometimes the simplest expressions of concern are the most meaningful. Speak from your heart and your sincere concern will be appreciated.

Here are some suggestions of supportive things to say:

- "Please let me know how I can help."
- "I'm not sure what to say, but I want you to know I care."
- "If you feel like talking, I'm here."
- "How are you doing today?"
- "I'm sorry to hear that you are going through this."
- "I'll keep you in my thoughts."
- When she looks good, tell her she's looking good!

The key here is to follow the lead of cancer patient.

Remember, your goal is to support her in whatever way she finds most comforting. *Sometimes just listening is the most helpful thing you can do.*

It is better to be honest and admit that you don't know what to say, than to simply stop calling or visiting out of fear of saying the wrong thing.

Your main objective should be to show concern and offer support. You can express encouragement, but resist the urge to be unrealistically optimistic.

Also, reducing the situation to a simple "stay positive" or "don't worry, everything will be ok" invalidates the person's very real fears, intense feelings and valid concerns.

There are a few things you should _avoid_ saying:

- "I know just what you should do"
- "I know just how you feel"
- "Don't worry"
- "I'm sure you'll be fine"
- "I feel helpless"
- "I don't know how you manage"
- "How much time do the doctors give you?"
- "You look pale"
- "You've lost so much weight"

The person is acutely aware of the changes in their appearance.

You don't need to point it out. _"It's good to see you"_ is a better way to greet her.

2: How to Be a Rock of Support

It's going to be very important that you step-up your emotional and physical strength level.

Without sounding trite, "Be a Rock" is a great way to describe the role you may need to take at this time.

Just remember that you can show strength for your loved one in many ways. You don't always have to present a chin-up, emotionless, stiff-upper-lip attitude.

Being a "rock" simply means remaining consistent in your behavior and support.

Cry with her, laugh with her, plan with her, do whatever she needs, but make sure you have your own support system in place too. Behind the scenes it's going to be a bumpy ride for everyone.

Being supportive does not mean you have to solve every problem. Sure, you want to make everything better, to give solutions to her problems, to help wash her pain away.

But this is a point in all of your lives where you're going to have to admit you're powerless in a lot of ways.

The solutions to the problems that are about to arise are going to be in the hands of many, many people.

Realize that while your loved one is going to need your help, *you* are going to need help too – and it's OK to ask others for help.

As much as we'd all like to think otherwise, we're not superheroes.

If you need a neighbor to bring in meals from time to time – ask them. If you need a ride – ask for it.

If you need a break – ask someone you trust to step-in.

If you need to take some time off from work – talk to your employer about the situation.

Maintaining your own support system is only one – albeit major – element to staying strong. This is a point where you're going to have to dig deep inside yourself and find what makes you strong.

You might find inner strength through prayer or a higher power, meditation, exercise, talking with others, or some other form of self-empowerment.

We will discuss these options in later chapters.

From the very beginning you will need to discover where your greatest source of strength lies and start exercising those muscles. Establish consistency.

3. Support Options for You as a Caretaker

You're going to be an amazing source of support for your friend or loved one.

During this ordeal, you also need to concentrate on the practices that are going to feed your own coping mechanisms and keep you emotionally stable and healthy.

As much as we'd like to believe it, we're not wells of boundless energy that can be tapped without replenishment.

You're going to need to be honest with yourself – and your loved one – about your own needs, and then take steps to make sure you're supported.

Call on Your Friends

If at all possible, call upon a friend who has been a caretaker for a loved one with cancer.

As we said in the introduction, cancer has touched most everyone's life in one way or another.

Even if you don't have direct contact with a person who has been in your shoes, it is highly likely a friend or an acquaintance will know someone who has.

When you find yourself in times of crisis or need, you're going to find that people will be there to help.

In general, the human race can be very supportive and will readily step up to bat when needed. You just have to be willing to ask!

You're going to find out who your friends are – and you will find that people will surprise you.

Support Groups

Make use of your contacts at the physician's office and ask them if they know of any support groups.

You need to be around people who have been where you are and where you're going, who can offer first-hand knowledge, support and encouragement.

While we like to think of ourselves as being very resourceful, you're embarking upon a journey into unknown territory.

Making use of the experience of the travelers before you will likely be one of your greatest resources.

Many people who care for cancer victims find a support group to be extremely helpful in reducing stress and staying emotionally stable.

Simply being able to talk with others who are going through the same things as you are can keep you from feeling so alone.

As a bonus, many of them will have already found ways to deal with the issues you're just now facing. Their advice and support can be a huge asset.

You can find support groups locally or online.

If you are in need of a therapist, your family doctor will be able to refer you to one.

Tap into Religion and Spirituality

If you're a person who believes in a form of religion or a higher power, make use of those beliefs.

Even if you do not follow a defined religion, there is a great source of untapped power when you give yourself over to the power of prayer.

Whatever form that takes for you, even if it's just acknowledging that there is a common source of energy everyone in the Universe shares, it can be comforting in times of stress.

The belief that faith heals has been around for centuries.

Long before there was any variation of formalized medicine, using ritualistic behavior and belief in a higher power to assist throughout the healing process was common practice.

You will not find any scientific evidence that faith will cause healing to occur.

What you will find is an overwhelming amount of information promoting the fact that giving yourself over to a higher power and the rituals you practice can help.

It will allow your stress levels to lessen, your overall sense of well-being to improve, and your anxiety levels to go down.

4: Staying Strong – Physically

There's going to be a lot of focus on your loved one: her health, her treatment, her lifestyle and all of the changes that occur in every area cancer touches.

Admittedly, this is where most of the focus should be.

Yet there will be times when you have to concentrate on yourself. Supporting a cancer patient throughout treatment and beyond is a difficult thing to do.

It's going to hit you in areas you never dreamed, both in your physical body and in your emotional health.

You need to be prepared for what is going to come at you. You must also realize that there is no way you can actually be 100% prepared.

You can do all the research, do all the reading, buck yourself up to take everything that is thrown at you, but until you're "in it", going through it, you really won't know what you're up against.

The best advice you can be given is to put your own strengthening practices in place early in the process.

Initiate practices that support your physical and emotional strengths with daily routines. This will allow your best self to shine through long-term.

Eat Healthy

Seems like a no-brainer, but maintaining a healthy lifestyle is one of your very best defenses at this point. When your body feels good, your physical and emotional health will fall into line as well.

Studies show that when people are under a lot of stress their bodies start to show physical damage.

It can start small with being forgetful and agitated or anxious and then move into larger, more serious symptoms such as aches and pains, diarrhea or nausea, even chest pains.

When you're under a lot of stress you may also experience behavioral problems, like sleeping too much or too little, or using alcohol and drugs to cope.

If you are noticing a lot of physical changes or issues cropping up, it might be helpful to keep a list of what you're eating, along with how you feel (see more about journaling in Chapter 5).

A daily food journal will show you at which times of the day you're most likely to reach for "junk food" or "comfort food".

If you're gaining or losing weight, a daily food journal will be indisputable evidence of where you need to focus on better nutrition.

You can look at your food journal from a few weeks prior and if you have noticed a shift in your weight, it's going to be easy to see what has led you there.

You'll easily see whether you're not eating enough in general, or you're not eating enough of the right foods.

After a few days, sit down and review what's been going on in your body and you may start to see some patterns.

You might notice that on the days you accompanied your loved one to chemo you felt nauseated.

You might see a connection between the Caesar salad you eat at the café on the corner on Wednesdays and the fact that, on Thursday night, you always have diarrhea.

Keeping a daily food journal is a practice many people find very useful, and you may want continue it throughout your life.

When you're concentrating on healthy eating and you've committed to writing down everything you eat during the day, chances are good you'll re-think the 5 Ding Dongs you just pulled out of the freezer. And of course, you'll feel better for it.

Exercise

Make sure you set aside some time to exercise. Exercising the body produces endorphins which naturally make you feel better.

It doesn't have to be a trip to the gym or strenuous exercise. Even getting outside and walking for 15 or 20 minutes will make a huge difference.

Be sure to talk with your physician before making any big changes in the exercise area. You should always make sure that what you're doing is safe for your body.

Sleep

Although it may seem like "common sense", getting enough quality sleep is essential for your physical and emotional wellbeing.

Whenever possible, try to stick to a regular sleep schedule. Going to bed at the same time each night will give you the best chance of getting a solid night's sleep.

Take a Multi Vitamin

Taking multivitamins can help to support your health and wellbeing throughout this stressful time.

To get the most benefit from a multivitamin/multi-mineral supplement, you must choose the right formula for you.

The B group vitamins are essential for the production of energy and also for the nervous system. These are especially beneficial during times of stress.

Magnesium, potassium and iron are also very important for maintaining your energy level.

Find a multi-vitamin, multi-mineral supplement that will help you support your health and stay strong.

Holding yourself accountable leads to healthy choices.

This in turn leads to a healthy body and increased strength – both physically and emotionally. That puts you in a position to be "The Rock" your loved one needs most.

5: Staying Strong – Emotionally

The most difficult part of this journey is the emotional one – learning how to cope. You're going to learn more about yourself in the upcoming months than you have in all your years past.

Even if your support role does not have a largely physical aspect to it (such as running to doctor's appointments and physically being present all the time) you still have to deal with the emotional toll this is going to take.

It's a good idea to immediately establish some patterns and practices to help support yourself emotionally. There's a lot going on in your life, so don't beat yourself up if you're not able to do everything. But take a look at the following tools and see which ones you might find helpful.

Journaling

It's going to be very important that you stay focused on your own personal health. Keep logs of how you feel, both physically and emotionally. If you don't currently keep a journal this might be a good time to start. You don't have to be a prolific writer to keep a journal. Simply writing down your thoughts and feelings has been proven to alleviate stress.

When you get up in the morning and before going to bed at night, take a few minutes to write a few sentences. Try to do this at the same time every day so you get into the habit.

Ask yourself, "How do I feel?" or "What happened today?" Ask yourself if there's anything in your body that feels different – or even that just doesn't feel quite right. If your back is aching or you have a headache, write it down.

Also note the days you feel good. If it's a day where you've had tons of energy and a positive attitude, write it down!

Journaling is a great way to take a step back and see the "big picture", which can be very therapeutic.

You can journal your feelings, emotions, stress levels, etc. You can also journal the physical influences on your mind and body. By journaling the food you eat and the amount of water you drink, you'll have a clear picture of your daily habits (the good and the not so good).

Keeping a daily/weekly food and water journal will be useful if you find yourself gaining or losing weight, experiencing an increase or decrease in physical pain, and many other food/hydration related indicators.

Organize Your Own Support Team

Organizing an informal support team of friends and relatives is a great way to get everyone involved.

There are online communities that offer tools to coordinate tasks among friends and caregivers. There are also online calendars that can be shared among the "support team" to help you organize activities, social visits and appointments.

If you're not a "computer person", you can buy a calendar at the dollar store and write in the various activities and commitments. Make sure the cancer patient has access to the calendar so she knows what to expect, who will be coming and when.

EFT (Emotional Freedom Technique)

EFT stands for "Emotional Freedom Technique." This is an extremely effective self-help method known as "Tapping" or "Meridian Tapping" that is used by hundreds of thousands of people all over the world.

Meridian Tapping has now gained much attention from many experts in the medical field. EFT is an innovative, non-invasive and drug-free approach to helping people achieve better health and well-being.

From treating chronic pain to helping people alleviate stress, EFT has been proven to work effectively and provide healing benefits.

There are many free videos on You Tube to give you an overview and working knowledge of EFT. It is safe, simple and easy to do and there is no equipment required.

Tapping is an effective tool for soothing or calming your body physically and your mind mentally or emotionally.

It is very empowering to be able to rely on yourself to bring calm to your mind and body, and to be able to do it anywhere, any time.

6. Escape through Meditation

Meditation can be one of the most useful tools in your arsenal.

You can use it to manage your stress levels and promote your overall well-being. Even five or ten minutes spent meditating each day can make a world of difference in your life.

The purpose of meditation will vary from person to person, but usually those who practice have a common goal: to quiet the mind, to relax, reflect and heal. All you really need is a quiet room and the intention to focus your energy for a few minutes.

The meditative process can open up a lot of feelings, especially if you're really taking the time to quiet the mind and focus inward.

Your meditative goals will change as your needs change, maybe even daily.

You can meditate specifically to channel your energy toward your loved one or you can meditate just to relax or to quiet your own mind.

If you're unsure of how to get started try these few simple exercises:

- Focus your attention on one thing, such as your breathing, an image, a word or a sound. *This is called a mantra*.

- Focus your attention on being only in the moment. Forget about everything else.

- When you exhale, intentionally let go of all the negativity of the day.

- On each inhalation concentrate on only calm, positive, passive feelings of gratitude.

- Let go of your worries for a few moments. Quiet your mind, focus on your mantra and breathe.

If you find your day is too busy you can meditate before going to bed. This is an amazing way to send yourself off into deep, rejuvenating sleep.

Lay in the dark, take long, deep breaths and relax every part of your body.

If you find you're unable to relax, try tightening/relaxing parts of your body.

Start with your toes – tighten, relax. Move to your calves – tighten, relax. Your thighs – tighten, relax.

By the time you've reached your forehead, every muscle in your body will be relaxed.

This is a great way to relieve the pent up tension you probably don't even realize you have.

Throughout the process, concentrate on breathing and allow your thoughts to only be on your mantra – the mantra can be that you want positive thoughts, to send healing to yourself, to allow yourself to calm, etc.

You will find that, when you're finished, your body will be much more relaxed and the stressors of the day will start to fall away.

7. Dealing with Your Dark Thoughts and Emotions

There's a lot coming at you all at once when you are caring for someone with cancer.

It's easy to run and hide, to live in denial of what is going on all around you. It's only human to subconsciously redirect your thoughts when there's something creeping in that you don't want to think about.

What if, in your mind, you're worried your loved one is going to die?

Your immediate response is to shove that down, to reassure yourself that they are not going to die and move on.

This is a normal, human response. But it's not necessarily the healthiest or most productive way to deal with dark thoughts.

Your self-protective instincts will kick-in when you start to think about something that's unpleasant.

What if you feel resentful because they got sick or because you have had to change your whole life to fit this new pattern cancer has caused?

You're probably going to beat yourself up about feeling that way. And then you're going to squash it down and repress those feelings. Again, this is a natural response.

The problem is that denying the dark thoughts that creep into your head will ultimately have negative consequences.

Those thoughts and worries will come out in some way eventually, whether it's lashing out at your family, physical manifestation (illness) in your body or forgetting to turn-in that big project at work… or eating five frozen Ding Dong's.

By allowing your thoughts to come out in a safe space you will counter-act some of the stress and strength-zapping consequences.

Throughout it all, remember that you're not going to get it "right" all the time. You're going to fall apart. You're going to do things wrong. You're going to say the wrong things and not always know how to say the right ones.

You're human and fallible. It's OK when that happens. Brush it off and move on.

Counseling

Your journal is going to be a huge help but it's not enough. If you don't currently talk with someone, such as a therapist or counselor, this is a good time to start.

While your journal is a safe space to acknowledge your feelings, it also doesn't respond to you.

Let's face it, sometimes that can be a good thing, but you might find you need someone who is trained in dealing with the emotions and stress a diagnosis like cancer can bring.

You're going to need coping skills and a safe space to vent, to cry, to laugh, to worry. Even if you've never talked with a therapist prior to this time, give it a try.

Consult with your insurance company to see what's available to you.

Many have limits on the length of treatment or the type of therapist you can see without a referral (psychologist vs. psychiatrist, for example).

Even one visit can help you learn some techniques for dealing with stress, how to cope and how to recognize when your body or subconscious mind is trying to tell you something.

You can talk with your loved one's primary physician or their oncologist if you're unsure where to find a therapist or if you're looking for one who specializes in cancer and caregivers.

They will likely have many counseling referral options for both you and your loved one.

Often times oncology offices are all-inclusive, offering these types of services alongside the physical treatment of the patient.

Go into therapy with an open mind and heart. Be honest, open and communicative to allow yourself to cope.

EFT (Emotional Freedom Technique)

As mentioned in a previous chapter, EFT (Meridian Tapping) is an effective tool for soothing or calming your body physically, and your mind mentally and emotionally.

EFT is free, easy to learn, requires no equipment and is very, very effective.

It is quite liberating to be able to rely on yourself, and not someone or something else, for calming yourself down and instantly getting back on track.

8. The Right Questions to Ask & When to Ask Them

You will find that there truly is great strength in knowledge.

From the minute the diagnosis is handed down start asking questions.

- What type of cancer is this?
- What stage of cancer is this?
- Where is the cancer?
- Has the cancer (metastasized) spread to other areas?
- Is this cancer treatable?
- If so, what is the treatment?
- What are the side effects of the treatment?
- Who do I call if I have problems?
  - When is it appropriate to call the doctor?
- Are there other options for treatment?
- How will this treatment affect the cancer?
- Will surgery be required?
- Where will the treatments occur (logistically)?
- If the cancer isn't treatable, what support options do we have?

- Is this cancer genetic?

• If it is genetic, should other family members be tested or concerned?

• What will insurance cover?

• What financial help is available?

Once you have put a "face" to the cancer start doing the research.

Get online and read, read, read.

Go to the library and read some more. Find books, not only on cancer treatment itself, but also self-help books to help support your loved one and yourself, your family and hers.

Consider looking into some therapy groups which will help further your support system.

There are typically many types of support groups available for just about any cancer scenario out there. With a quick Google search you should be able to find ones in your area.

What you find is going to be scary.

You're going to find stories of success and stories of tragedy.

You're going to find people who have gone through treatment smoothly and easily and you're going to find people whose lives have become a living hell.

You will find life and you will find death.

Try to keep it all in perspective and stay as neutral as possible.

Remember that you have just begun. As the doctor will tell you, every person is different.

Every cancer is different. Every treatment plan is different.

All you can do is gather as much information as you can so that you can help make informed decisions later.

You will have a flood of information coming at you during all of this, so don't expect to take it all in all at once.

Do try to stay organized.

- You might want to take notes or print out or photocopy important items.

- Consider keeping it all in a binder that you can take with you to appointments.

- You can also have the binder handy when you're on the phone with insurance companies, hospitals, and other organizations.

We will discuss this in more detail in Chapter 10.

Read all you can about the type of cancer you're dealing with and anything that may arise as a result.

Keep an eye out for potential treatment options and possible consequences of those treatment options. Know what to do and who to turn to when you're faced with problems.

If your loved one is facing chemotherapy or radiation, read about the different types of chemo and the side effects that occur.

Surgery might not have the same long-term side effects, but comes with its own risks. Find out what the accepted treatment is, and what to expect from each treatment option.

Remember: Knowledge is Power!

You will feel stronger – and, in effect, be stronger and cope better – when you're well-armed with information.

The unknown is scary, so try to eliminate as much of the unknown as possible.

9. What to Do Legally

There are going to be times when your loved one needs someone to advocate for her.

If you're a spouse or next of kin who will be responsible for talking with doctors and other health care providers, being there during treatment/procedures, even helping with billing or talking to the insurance companies, you're going to need some documentation to back you up.

Make sure you and your loved one have a clear plan of how she wants things to be handled.

This might be a tough conversation to have, but it's a necessary one.

And do it immediately, don't wait.

This isn't a conversation that should be put off even for a moment.

And most certainly it should be had before ANY treatment options are undertaken.

If you're the next of kin you must know her wishes – how she wants to be treated, how she wants her life and well-being handled in the event something goes wrong, and any living will or "Do Not Resuscitate" (DNR) directives, if applicable.

You may need to become her voice if she is no longer able to communicate, and you need to be legally able to do so on her behalf.

Part of being an advocate requires open communication, not just with your loved one but also with her care providers.

Her doctors must know her wishes, stated in writing, in a clear manner, with documents drafted by a legal professional.

This is especially important if you're the next of kin that may not be recognized legally by the state, such as if you're in a same-sex relationship or are "family" in name only, but not by blood.

Every pertinent family member should be given copies of legal documents as they apply to them, along with a copy to be kept with the family lawyer.

These documents should be readily available in the event a situation warrants.

Here is an example:

You and your partner are same sex, and legally married in Vermont. Unfortunately your union is not considered a legal marriage in the state of Nevada where you are on vacation together.

Your partner, who is undergoing cancer treatment, has collapsed and has been admitted into the ICU. The ICU doctors do not want to allow you to participate in her treatment.

They will not allow you to make decisions and are not legally bound to do so. However, if you have paperwork showing your legal connection and the fact you're her Power of Attorney (POA) they *must* allow you to participate as the directives show.

Additionally, since you have all the paperwork from start to finish: lab results, doctor's names, pathology reports, and treatment plans – when they ask for it, you've got it with you in your binder – she will be able to get the care she needs without the added delay or worry that something is missed.

Being an advocate for a cancer patient can take many different forms.

It can mean being present during treatments and, when you see something that's alarming, or a procedure being done with which you're unfamiliar, standing up to ask questions.

Being an advocate means you must have a voice when the patient does not and means you have to be the eyes, ears and voice for the patient first. Ask questions – A LOT of questions.

An important thing to remember about being an advocate is that you do not impose upon the privacy of your loved one.

She is the boss and has entrusted you to advocate for her. Don't abuse that trust.

You don't have to take on a raging bull stance. You can be a strong, effective advocate and do so in a polite yet firm manner. You can be an advocate without offending and alienating her medical providers.

Keep communicating, asking her what she wants and needs for you to do, and above all else, respect her wishes.

Speaking of wishes, one other important area where the patient needs support is regarding her final wishes.

Talking about wills, DNR (Do Not Resuscitate) orders, and funeral plans is never easy – even with a healthy person.

No one likes to face his or her own mortality, but when someone is faced with a potentially terminal diagnosis, it's a crucial conversation.

The reality is that people die from cancer every day.

*People **recover** every day too.*

You can greatly reduce the stress of everyone involved by helping your loved one put her affairs in order *before* undergoing any sort of treatment.

Remember, you're not saying "you're going to die."

You're simply taking one more worry away.

10. How to Organize the Mountain of Paperwork

The mountain of paperwork that engulfs a cancer patient is overwhelming – and often completely unexpected.

There will be dozens of forms to fill out, medical history to be researched and repeated over and over again, financial statements, lists of medications, and every new health care provider on the team will want his or her own copy.

Expect to deal with a primary care physician, an oncologist, an endocrinologist, a radiologist, a chemotherapy specialist, social workers, case managers, nurse practitioners, physical therapists…and the list goes on. Just keeping up with the paperwork can seem like a full time job.

If your loved one is covered by insurance you will need to work with her doctors and insurance billing departments …
a lot.

Some insurance companies are notorious for making things difficult, so it's going to be very important that you keep everything organized.

Being able to produce a specific piece of paper when it's needed can mean the difference between the insurance covering the cost of treatment, and your loved one paying out of pocket.

Radiation treatments alone can total thousands of dollars per week, so staying organized is vital.

First, you'll want to collect information from the doctors.

When the diagnosis comes down, get it in writing. When the treatment plan is recommended by the physician, get it in writing.

If the physician has recommended you seek a second opinion, get it in writing. When you get the second opinion, *get their recommendations in writing*.

For example, say you've gotten the second opinion, however the insurance company is rejecting the claim.

They're citing it not necessary to see that specialist. You will have the recommendation from the primary physician already in-hand and ready to fax to the insurance company.

Imagine how many calls – and hours – you've saved simply by having the necessary paperwork to back you up!

Here's another example: The insurance company doesn't want to pay for a specific treatment option.

You, however have two letters in your trusty binder; one from the primary physician and one of the second physician's opinion, and both letters recommend the same course of treatment.

Since you have this in-hand, you'll be able to fax it off to the insurance company and get it seen by the review board much more quickly than if you had to wait for the letter to be generated from both doctors' offices, sent to you and/or faxed to the insurance company's review board.

Keep every bill, every receipt, and every letter.

Keep them all organized by date, type of document and by physician.

This will be helpful down the road when you need to advocate for procedures the insurance company may try to weasel out of paying.

Don't let this chapter scare you. You may have a perfectly easy insurance process all the way throughout, but you cannot bank on that – literally – so you want to be prepared just in case.

Insurance companies like to reject claims. It's how they do things, so be prepared to work for the financial reimbursement.

Keeping organized while coping with cancer will get easier as you go along. The recommendation to "keep everything" doesn't mean you need to cart it all around to every doctor's appointment.

There are, however, some items you should have with you at all times:

- Patient Identification
- Insurance Card
- Medic Alert bracelet

You may also be required to show proof of a referral if you're seeing a new doctor or getting a new procedure. In this case, make sure you have the letter of referral from the originating physician to present to the new doctor.

Conclusion

We've talked a lot about communication. This is at the heart of many of the topics that have been discussed throughout this guide.

Communication is at the heart of most things in life really. It will be the greatest tool you have throughout your life, and in helping your friend or loved one through this dark time in her life.

Talking with your loved one, talking with her physicians and support staff, talking with yourself, talking with those who will be supporting you – the heart of the matter is going to lie in being honest, open and communicative from beginning to end.

However you choose to offer support, know that you have so many who have come before you, who have been in your shoes, who have experienced everything you're about to go through.

Coping with cancer when someone you love is diagnosed is not a process you have to go through alone. Use the resources you have available to you as they are boundless.

You are not alone in this experience and *you will get through it*.

About the Author

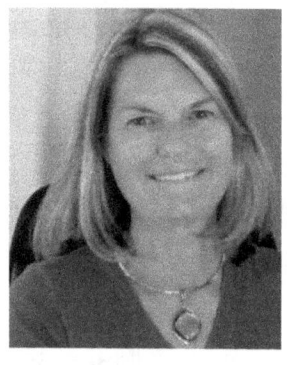

Donna Bainton has been an author, speaker and naturopathic consultant since 1990.

She is the founder of Begin Within Online Academy, where she teaches women how to solve their health issues using holistic solutions.

Programs range from laser focused 1-hour micro-courses and 7-day challenges, to a 52-week long Ultimate Holistic Health Course.

On her action-oriented blog _DonnaBainton.com_, you'll find enlightening articles and free resources on topics such as anti-aging, health, mindset, pain and weight management.

Donna is known for her natural health and inspirational books and courses, transformational workshops, online coaching programs and live events.

Additional Resources

BeginWithinOnlineAcademy.com

DonnaBainton.com

Copyrights

ISBN-13: 978-1539855033

ISBN-10: 1539855031

Limits of Liability and Disclaimer of Warranty

This publication is designed to provide accurate and authoritative information in regard to the subject matter covered.

The ideas, suggestions and procedures in this book are not intended as a substitute for the medical advice of a trained health care professional.

All matters regarding health, healing, nutrition and wellness require medical supervision.

Consult your physician or health care provider before adopting the suggestions in this book. Also consult your physician or health care provider about any condition that may require diagnosis, treatment or medical attention.

The author and publisher shall not be liable for your misuse of this material. This book is strictly for informational, educational, inspirational and entertainment purposes.

www.ingramcontent.com/pod-product-compliance
Lightning Source LLC
Chambersburg PA
CBHW070239290526
45789CB00004B/1693